NEUROLOGY - LABORATORY AND CLINICAL RESEARCH DEVELOPMENTS

NEUROPLASTICITY FOLLOWING SKILL AND STRENGTH TRAINING

NEUROLOGY - LABORATORY AND CLINICAL RESEARCH DEVELOPMENTS

Additional books in this series can be found on Nova's website under the Series tab.

Additional E-books in this series can be found on Nova's website under the E-books tab.

NEUROLOGY - LABORATORY AND CLINICAL RESEARCH DEVELOPMENTS

NEUROPLASTICITY FOLLOWING SKILL AND STRENGTH TRAINING

ALAN J. PEARCE

AND

DAWSON J. KIDGELL

Nova Biomedical
Nova Science Publishers, Inc.
New York

For permission to use material from this book please contact us:
Telephone 631-231-7269; Fax 631-231-8175
Web Site: http://www.novapublishers.com

Additional color graphics may be available in the e-book version of this book.

LIBRARY OF CONGRESS CATALOGING-IN-PUBLICATION DATA

Pearce, Alan J., 1969-
Neuroplasticity following skill and strength training / Alan J. Pearce and Dawson J. Kidgell.
p. ; cm.
Includes bibliographical references and index.
ISBN 978-1-61728-762-6 (softcover)
1. Neuroplasticity. 2. Motor learning. 3. Physical education and training. I. Kidgell, Dawson J. II. Title.
[DNLM: 1. Neuronal Plasticity. 2. Resistance Training. 3. Transcranial Magnetic Stimulation. WL 102]
QP363.3.P43 2010
612.8'11--dc22

2010025939

Published by Nova Science Publishers, Inc. † New York

CONTENTS

PREFACE

The ability for the human motor cortex to change based on experience is now well accepted. Termed neuroplasticity, convincing evidence is available to challenge the long held view of a functionally stable neocortex that is unable to change. The aim of this text is to provide data collected in our laboratory, by us and in collaboration with others, using the technique of transcranial magnetic stimulation (TMS), as evidence of neuroplasticity following short and long term skill and strength training. Short-term skill training studies have shown significant increases in corticospinal excitability (12%) projecting to an intrinsic hand muscle (first dorsal interosseous, FDI) during the performance of a simple fine motor task associated with greater degree of precision compared to an identical but less difficult task. These findings have been reproduced in both anisometric (ramped) and dynamic visuomotor tracking tasks (in FDI) with corticospinal excitability increased during both slow and precise anisometric and dynamic tasks (increases of 42% and 56% respectively), compared to the same tasks being performed fast and rhythmically. Neuroplasticity has also been demonstrated in individuals who have practiced complex motor skills over long-periods of time. Using the technique of TMS mapping, allowing for the construction of topographical maps, we investigated the representation of the FDI in Olympic badminton athletes. In comparison to sub-elite competitive players and control subjects, Olympic athletes showed increased corticospinal excitability and alterations in the map representation suggesting functional reorganisation following long-term motor practice. Strength exercise has been considered a form of motor skill training and for this reason we have also investigated neural adaptations following short-term strength training. Four weeks of maximal isometric strength training in the FDI demonstrated a significant increase in strength (34%) and changes in corticospinal inhibition (seen as a reduction in the cortical silent period of 25 ms). Similar increases in strength (28%) were observed following four weeks unilateral training of the biceps brachii muscle, however, neural adaptations were reflected in greater corticospinal excitability rather than corticospinal inhibition. In a second part of the same study, we also found significant increases in strength (19%) and corticospinal excitability projecting to the biceps brachii muscle in the contralateral untrained limb, in the absence of muscular hypertrophy in either arm. The studies presented in this text has extended on previous research, however by using TMS we are able to provide evidence of neuroplastic changes in the human central nervous system, in relation to motor skill and strength training.

Chapter 1

INTRODUCTION

The ability for the human primary motor cortex (M1) to adapt and reorganise, based on experience and/or training, is now accepted and ubiquitously termed neuroplasticity. With evidence collected from a range of non-invasive neuro-imaging techniques, to challenge the long held view of a functionally stable neocortex immutable to change, investigations now focus on the degree and variations in the forms of neuroplasticity following experience or training interventions [1].

Neuroplasticity in humans has been demonstrated across a range of conditions, including acute sensory and peripheral manipulations, such as electrical stimulation [2], amputation [3], nerve deafferentation or anaesthesia [4]. Reorganisation in topographical representation, providing evidence of experience dependant neuroplasticity, have been shown in neurological conditions such as stroke [5], dystonia [6], Parkinson's disease [7] and multiple sclerosis [8].

Neural adaptations have also been demonstrated following training interventions such as motor skill acquisition and strength training. We have used the technique of transcranial magnetic stimulation (TMS) to investigate neural adaptations and functional reorganisation following fine motor skill performance, long-term motor skill training, short-term strength training, and cross-education to the untrained limb following unilateral strength training. This has been the focus of the research in our laboratory and will form the basis of this text. We will briefly describe the technique of TMS before the presentation of these studies.

TRANSCRANIAL MAGNETIC STIMULATION (TMS)

It is possible to study the brain using electromagnetic stimulation. Non invasive brain stimulation, particularly TMS, was first developed in 1985 [9]. Commercially available stimulators (Fig 1) suitable for human study have been available since the middle 1980s with minimal risk to healthy individuals [10]. Although quite rare, individuals may experience mild local discomfort on the scalp musculature or a headache. However, since the introduction of commercially available single pulse stimulators, only three reported cases of seizure have been reported in adult patients with large cerebral infarcts or other lesions, with no adverse reports in healthy adults [10] or children [11,12], making single pulse TMS very safe [13,14].

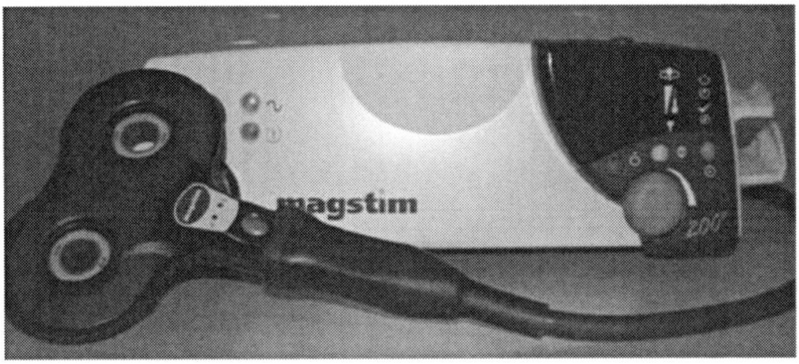

Figure 1. Magstim 200^2 single pulse stimulator with a 'figure of eight' magnetic coil. The figure of eight coil contains two small magnets in reverse polarity enabling a more focused electromagnetic impulse than the standard circular coil (from author's own image collection).

The mechanisms and principles of TMS are well covered in reviews by Hallet [13, 14]. However, briefly, TMS employs time varying magnetic fields that induce electrical currents in conductive neural tissue, with the induced electric field being proportional to the rate of the magnetic field. If the current induced by the electric field is of sufficient amplitude and duration, it will depolarise neural tissue, recorded and measured as a motor evoked potential (MEP) in the surface electromyogram (sEMG) of the target muscle. There are several quantifiable components with TMS. The motor threshold (MT) being the minimum amount of stimulation required to produce a MEP. The MT may be observed in both resting muscle or during a tonic voluntary contraction, and may be termed active motor threshold or AMT [15]. The measurable components of a MEP are illustrated in Figure 2: latency; MEP amplitude; and silent period duration. The latency of the

MEP is a reproducible measure of the corticospinal conduction time and measured from the time of stimulation to the onset of the MEP [13,14]. For example, it is well known that conduction time from stimulation to a hand muscle is approximately 20 ms of which Hess et al. [16] estimated that approximately 13 ms is from peripheral mechanisms with the remaining time comprising central conduction, synaptic delay at the motoneuron and conduction down a short intradural segment of the motor root [17]. Further, it is also well known that tonic voluntary activation can reduce the corticomotor conduction time of an average of 2 – 3 ms [18] due to facilitation of spinal motoneurons.

The MEP is a relatively synchronous muscle response that can be measured on the sEMG [13, 14]. The amplitude of a MEP is influenced by inhibitory and excitatory interconnections descending on the motor neurone pool at the time of stimulation [19] and is usually quantified by measuring the peak to peak amplitude of the MEP "spike" waveform on the sEMG (see Fig 2). Similar to latency, facilitation of a muscle will reduce the threshold for a MEP to occur, lowering the intensity of stimulation applied to the participant. Individuals respond differently to TMS, that is the MEP response for similar stimulus intensity between individuals will differ in amplitude [20]. However, when controlled for torque and type of motor task, the MEP is a reliable intra-partipant measure [21, 22], allowing for confident interpretation of changes following acute or chronic interventions. However, it is not uncommon to see investigators using a MEP/M-wave ratio to normalise individual MEP variations between participants [23].

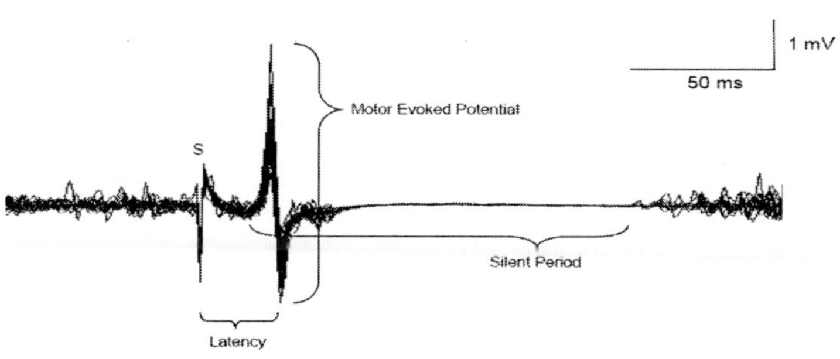

Figure 2. The components of a MEP as recorded on sEMG. Overlayed image of 30 sweeps, obtained from the first dorsal interosseous (FDI) muscle following TMS over the contralateral motor cortex, illustrating the reliability of the MEP when the muscle is controlled for contraction level. The MEP is visible approximately 20-25 ms following cortical stimulation (S). This is termed latency. MEP amplitude is calculated by cursoring the peak to peak value of the MEP. Silent period (SP) is measured by cursoring onset of MEP to return of sEMG activity (Image from [24]).

In facilitated muscle contractions, the MEP will be preceded by a distinctive period of sEMG non activity, termed the silent period or SP (Fig 2). The SP can last anywhere between 50 ms to 300 ms following stimulation, and provides a measure of the strength of inhibition in the corticospinal pathway [25, 26]. It is now recognised that the SP arises from a combination of subcortical (spinal cord) and cortical inhibition [14, 27] and with single pulse TMS the duration of the silent period is thought to reflect γ-aminobutyric acid ($GABA_b$) mediated inhibitory processes [28].

The SP has been shown to correlate with MEP [29], despite the evidence that the SP represents different aspect of cortical excitability [26, 30] It is well recognised that the SP will be recruited at lower levels of stimulation, including below AMT [31], and saturate earlier than the MEP [29].

Experimental and clinical studies have shown that the SP can be altered. Hess et al [32] has demonstrated task-dependant changes in SP duration of various tasks. During tactile exploration of a small object, SP duration was longer than for an isometric contraction. Conversely, SP duration was shortened during visuomotor tasks compared to the isometric contraction. Clinical studies of individuals with neurological conditions have shown reduced SP in Parkinson's disease, thought to be due to decreased effectiveness of cortical inhibitory inputs following TMS [33]. Conversely, lengthening of the SP has been shown in epilepsy patients [34] and in stroke patients [35] with these authors suggesting that the SP lengthening was due to a reduced drive of afferent signals to the M1. For further information on evoked potentials (latency, MEP and SP) from TMS, the reader is directed to Hallet [13,14], Pascual-Leone et al [36], Boniface & Ziemann [37], and Wasserman et al [20].

TMS Compared to Other Neuroimaging Techniques

A major difference between neuroimaging techniques, such as functional magnetic resonance imaging (fMRI), and TMS is that TMS has the ability to show excitation and inhibition of the corticospinal pathway, thereby demonstrating an area's direct influence on a motor performance. There are a number of studies that have directly shown increased excitability [38, 39] in a cortical motor area during task activation or, conversely, using TMS to transiently suppress regions of the cerebral cortex, providing stronger evidence of motor regions directly involved in a task [40]. It is for this reason that TMS has been pivotal in a variety of research areas within neurophysiology and motor control. Furthermore, many studies now combine both spatial imaging of techniques such as fMRI with temporal techniques such as TMS to investigate areas of the brain directly involved with motor function [41, 42].

TMS also has the ability to be used as a neuroimaging tool, illustrating topographical representation of muscles on the motor cortex in healthy [26], athletic [43] or, conversely, individuals who have suffered a neurological condition [5, 7]. Using a methodology based on a latitude and longitude system, TMS can be employed to stimulate a number of areas overlying the motor cortex systematically (Fig 3a). Averaging the MEP waveforms collected over each site (Fig 3b), a topographical matrix of MEP vs stimulus site can be generated to provide a representation of the muscle targeted during stimulation. An example of a map calculated from the topographical matrix is presented in Figure 3c. For an in depth discussion on the technique and methodology of TMS mapping, the reader is directed to Wilson et al [26] or Thickbroom & Mastaglia [44].

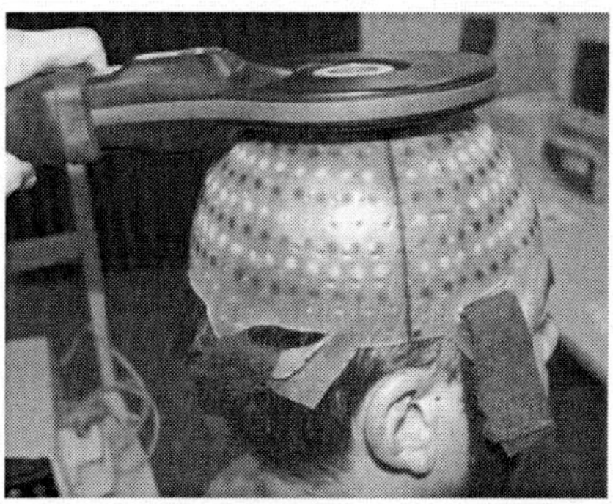

a

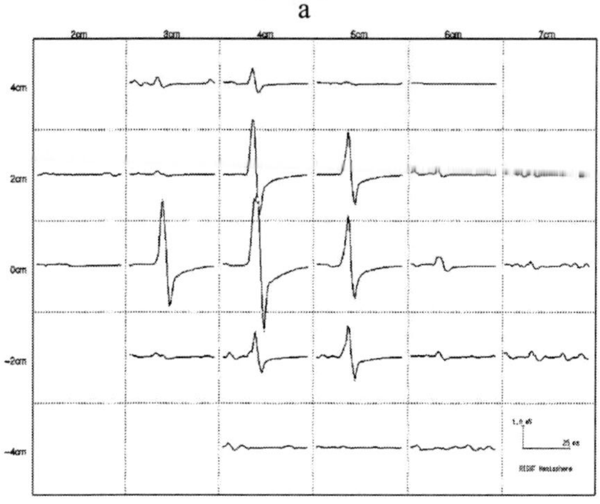

B

Figure Continued

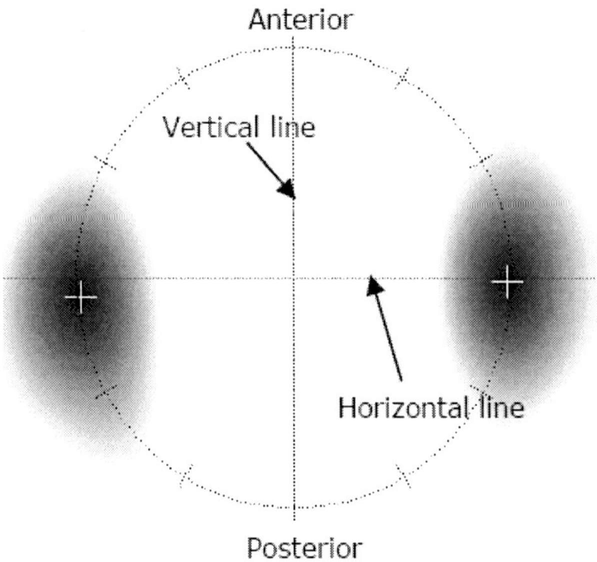

c

Figure 3a – c. Methodology of TMS mapping developed by Wilson et al [26]. Participants wear a snug fitted cap (a) with markings of 1 cm distance in both antero-posterior (A-P) and medio-lateral (M-L) directions. TMS is delivered at sites approximately in the motor area for the target muscle. The optimal site is where the largest MEP is identified and then as the coil is moved away from this site in A-P and M-L directions, the MEP reduces in size until no waveform can be identified. Figure 3b illustrates topographic MEP wave forms for one hemisphere. The mean of four stimuli at each site, calculated and plotted as a function of scalp site stimulated to create a representation of the muscle on a 2-D surface (c). The white cross represents the centre of the maps and the circular dotted line represented 62 mm from the vertical mid-line (images from [24] and authors own collection).

Chapter 2

NEURAL ADAPTATIONS FOLLOWING MOTOR SKILL TRAINING

Neural adaptations may occur at a number of sites within the neuromuscular pathway [45]. Changes may be as a result of strength training, but may also be the result of skill training, as it has been argued that strength training and skill training are closely connected in terms of adaptations occurring by similar mechanisms originating in the cerebral cortex [46]. This section of the text will present research from our laboratory, and in collaboaration with others, investigating neuro-muscular responses following precision movement and long-term skill acquisition.

SHORT-TERM SKILL TASK STUDIES

There have been a number of TMS studies, performed in the 1990s, investigating the neural adaptations of the human motor system, with many of these studies using dynamic movement paradigms such as comparison of simple (single joint) versus complex (multi-joint) movement tasks [47, 48], or comparison of corticospinal changes between 'precision' ('grip' and 'push') isometric tasks to 'power' ('grasp' and 'load/hold') isometric tasks [49].

Taken together, these studies [47-49] indicate that cortical activity changes are reflective of movement tasks requiring increased demand on the neuromuscular system. However, although these studies have compared similar muscle groups and levels of sEMG activity, the tasks performed differed. Therefore, we conducted two studies investigating corticospinal parameters of MEP latency and amplitude, and SP duration during the performance of *similar* motor tasks, at *similar* levels of muscular activation but differing in the difficulty of precision in successfully performing the tasks.

The first study [50] required ten participants (20 to 45 years; 3 female, 7 male) to abduct the first index finder of their preferred hand, activating the first dorsal interosseous muscle (FDI), against a force transducer mounted on a specifically-designed board. Participants (two visits to the laboratory, one week apart) were instructed to hold a static contraction at 10 (± 3%) of maximum voluntary contraction (MVC) sEMG against the force transducer, providing visuomotor feedback via a computer monitor displaying markers that the participants response marker needed to be maintained within. The display showed the participant's response marker reflecting changes in static force between two stationery marker bars. During the "easy" static task, force variations would be presented accurately. However during the "difficult" static task, adjustments made by the participant would cause a greater amplification in the position of the marker, making the task more difficult to control. The participant was not informed of the order of tasks which were randomized between participants.

TMS was delivered of 40 stimuli in eight sets of five stimuli, 10 s apart and 30 s rest between each set, during performance of these tasks, using TMS techniques described earlier in chapter 1. No differences were observed in MEP latency ("difficult" 20.8 ± 0.7 ms vs "easy" 20.6 ± 0.9 ms; p=0.41) or SP duration ("difficult" 105.70 ± 21.22 ms vs "easy" 107.60 ± 18.65 ms; p=0.16). However, MEP amplitude was observed to be 12% larger for the "difficult" task (4.91± 2.69 mV) compared to the "easy" task (4.39 ± 2.66 mV; p=0.04).

The second study [51] continued investigations using the same paradigm of precision motor tasks. However, in two studies (with 12 participants; 5 male and 7 female, 20-38 years), we compared the effect of increasing the precision of the task using dynamic movement. Study I ("Force Tracking"), we used the same force transducer to the previous study [50], with participants instructed to control their response cursor by using anisometric (ramped) movement, applying or releasing pressure to move their response cursor in an upward or downward direction on the computer monitor. Study II ("Position Tracking") incorporated a dial potentiometer with participants controlling their cursor whilst holding a pincer grip and moving the dial in an anti-clockwise (facilitating abduction of the first finger) or clockwise (adduction of first finger) fashion, to move the cursor up or down on the monitor. Visuomotor tasks were conducted at similar levels of force (10 ± 3% of MVC EMG) at two speeds: "slow" being one tracking cycle of up and down in 10 s; and "fast" being two tracking cycles in 10 s. Corticospinal changes where observed (an example is presented in Fig 4) with significant increases (p=0.002) in excitability demonstrated during slow speed tasks in Study I (42.3 ± 16.8%) and Study II (56.3 ± 34.2%). Moreover, a significant reduction (p=0.001) in corticospinal inhibition was also observed during both tracking tasks at slow (59.3 ± 13.7%) and fast speeds (31.9 ± 12.3%).

The data presented in these two studies, illustrates the ability of the corticospinal system to alter in response to the demands of a motor task. It would be remiss to suggest that these two studies suggest neural adaptations or neuroplasticity occurring, given the immediacy of the response to the task requirement; however the findings demonstrate the value of challenging the corticospinal system during motor task performance, which with repeated bouts can induce neuroplasticity.

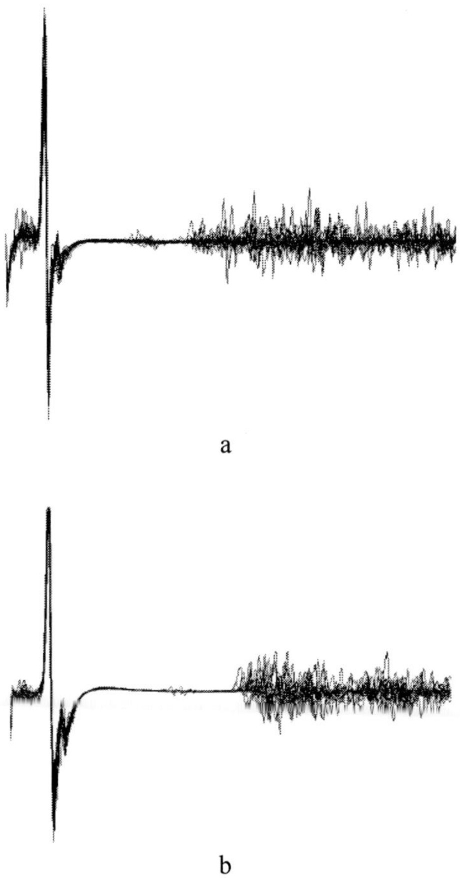

Figure 4. Example of raw data from one participant of 40 overlaid stimuli, with similar sEMG activation levels, showing increased MEP amplitude (6.9 to 5.7 mV) and reduced SP duration (115 vs 151 ms) between the slow (a) and fast (b) visuomotor tracking task [51].

LONG-TERM SKILL TRAINING

Further to rapid alterations in excitability and/or inhibition during motor tasks requiring precision, the corticospinal pathway is also responsive following skill acquisition. Pascual-Leone and colleagues [38, 39] presented convincing evidence, using TMS, that the cortical representation of muscles on the M1 can change rapidly following repeated practice. These findings have been supported by research using other neuroimaging techniques such as fMRI [52, 53].

However, despite considerable discussion in the expertise literature regarding the time requirements to become an expert at a skill, e.g. 10,000 hours or 10 years practice [54], little is known about the neurophysiological responses underlying extensive practice. Elbert and colleagues' [55] well cited magnetoencephalography study showed alterations in sensory representation for the fingering digits of violin players but not for the digits of the bow hand, indicating that a long-lasting change in the sensory cortex had occurred in response to the repetitive practice and performance. However, our study [43] investigated the corticomotor representation of a hand muscle in a group of highly skilled elite racket athletes, comparing representation to those in a group of competitive (but not elite) players, and a group of controls, who had never regularly played any racket sport.

Studies were performed on ten badminton players: five elite athletes (4 male, 1 female; 22-28 years) all who regularly competed at Olympic and international level and trained for an average duration of 21.6 hours per week; and five non-elite recreational competitive players (3 male, 2 female; 22-50 years) who played regularly (three times per week) but did not specifically train their skills. All but one player (in the elite group) were right handed. Ten participants (5 male, 5 female; 23-40 years) who did not participate in any form of racket sport, served as controls.

TMS mapping technique, briefly described in Chapter 1 [26], for the representation of the FDI muscle was used, generating maps shown in Figure 5a-c. Maps generated for the control participants (Fig 5a) and non-elite players (Fig 5b) showed symmetrical placement (centre of maps located between 55-63 mm lateral to the vertical line) of within 3 mm, regardless of handedness or playing hand. However significant displacement (between 5-16 mm; $p=0.02$) in the maps projecting to the playing hand in the elite players was observed with centre of maps ranging between 39-59 mm for the playing hand. It should be noted that the displacement in the maps were in both directions; in three elite athletes, maps were shifted medially in three players (athletes 2, 3 & 5) and laterally in the remaining two players (athletes 1 & 4). Not presented in the study, but of interest no less, was that the left handed elite player, athlete 5 (Fig 5c), considered himself as right-hand dominant for all other tasks [56], apart from badminton.

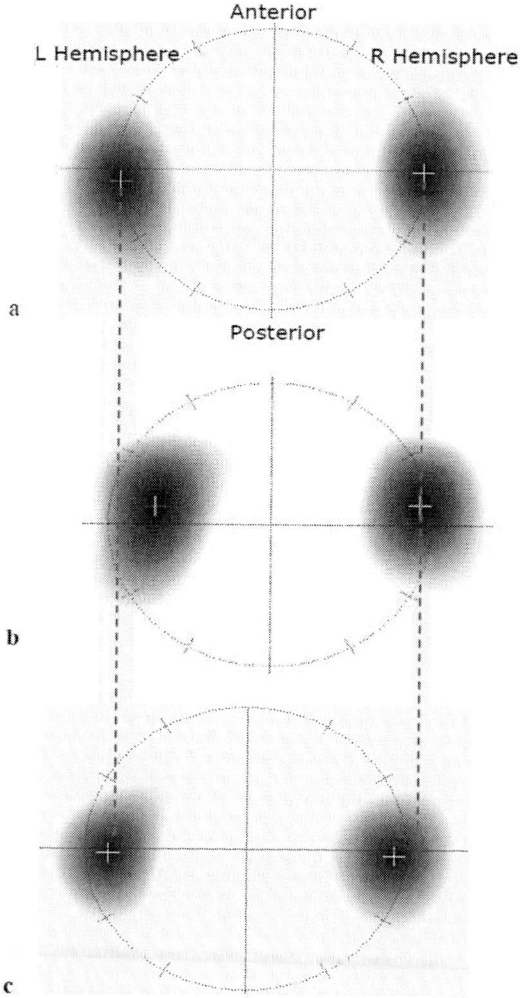

Figure 5. Corticomotor representation of FDI muscle on both hemispheres for a recreational badminton player (a), and athletes 1 (b) and 5 (c). The center of the maps is indicated by a white cross (+) and the circular dotted line represents 62 mm from the vertex. Note interhemispheric symmetry in the control participant map (a) and dotted line for athletes' non-playing hand lies similar to the control participant. Asymmetrical maps were observed for all athletes; the map for right handed athlete 1 (b) shows medial shifting of the left hemisphere and the map for left handed athlete 5 (c) shows medial shifting for right hemisphere [43].

Although no correlation was found between the amount of map displacement to the athletes' onset of formal training or the amount of practice at the time of the study, the findings from this study provide evidence of plasticity in corticomotor reorganisation in response to long-term, structured, effective motor skill reinforcement. This is supported by the maps from the non-elite players. Despite regular play by the non-elite players, and being skilful in their own right, these players did not undertake skilled practice sessions such as that of the athlete group, where repetition was a feature of elite training, further supporting the importance of specific motor training in improving skills.

Chapter 3

NEURAL ADAPTATIONS FOLLOWING SHORT-TERM STRENGTH TRAINING

Neural mechanisms have been speculated to account for increases in strength, particularly in the first four weeks of a strength training program where there is a noticeable absence of muscular hypertrophy [57]. There are a number of proposed neural mechanisms underpinning strength improvements which include peripheral adaptations such as changes in motor unit behaviour, reduced co-contraction of antagonist muscle groups; and increased descending drive from supraspinal centres, and modifications in spinal cord circuitry, such as increased motor neuron excitability. For further discussion on these proposed mechanisms the reader is directed to reviews by Semmler and Enoka [45], and Folland and Williams [58]. There have also been hypotheses offered that neural mechanisms underpinning strength and skill improvements are controlled by similar mechanisms originating in the cerebral cortex [46, 59]. These hypotheses have been directly related to neural mechanisms underpinning cross-education strength and skill changes; however, there may also be a basis to suggest that strength training is a form of skill training [60, 61]. Despite extensive discussion on the role of the nervous system in short-term strength changes [45, 58], limited evidence on specific corticospinal mechanisms has been presented. Moreover, studies that have used TMS have shown contradictory findings with two studies [62, 63] reporting no change in MEP amplitudes post-training whilst studies by Griffen and Cafarelli [64] and Beck et al [65] showed increased MEP amplitudes following short term strength training. These differences may be attributed to differing training regimes, resistance loads and muscles used, illustrating the need for further investigation.

Research in our laboratory has aimed to extend on these initial findings. In particular, studies have focused on quantifying the corticospinal responses following acute (four weeks) strength training in a hand muscle and forearm flexor muscles. We have also measured corticospinal changes in the contralateral arm following unilateral short-term strength training.

Short-Term Strength Training of Hand and Upper Limb Muscles

The first study [66] investigated the acute corticospinal responses following isometric strength training of the FDI muscle. Sixteen healthy, right-handed participants (24.12 ± 5.21 years) were randomly allocated to either a strength training (7 males, 1 female) or a control group (6 males, 2 females). Participants assigned to the strength training group completed 12 supervised strength training sessions over a four week training period that involved 6 sets of 10 repetitions of 3 s static holds, with a 3 s rest, against a force transducer, with 3 min rest between sets. TMS evoked MEPs (described earlier) and M-waves (delivered with supramaximal electrical stimulation of the ulnar nerve) were applied prior to and following the strength training intervention at 10% above AMT during a constant static contraction of 5% and 20% MVC.

Mean strength in the training group increased 34% ($p=0.01$). Normalised as a percentage of the maximum M-wave, there were no significant differences in the size of the MEP between groups at 5% of MVC (trained group 8.6% increase versus control 2.7% decrease, $p=0.47$) and 20% MVC (9.7% increase versus 0.3% decrease, $p=0.21$). However, following strength training, the duration of the SP was significantly decreased in the strength training group. Specifically, at 5% MVC there was a 16 ms reduction ($p=0.01$) in the trained group (145 ± 18 ms to 129 ± 38 ms) compared to the control group (133 ± 51 ms to 124 ± 27 ms) and at 20% MVC there was a 25 ms reduction ($p=0.03$) in the trained group (pre 129 ms ± 34 ms to post 104 ± 29 ms) compared to the control group (pre 126 ms ± 10.5 ms to post 129 ± 11 ms). Correlation analysis showed a moderate negative correlation between the change in strength and the mean change in SP duration ($r=-0.51$, $p=0.05$) for the strength training group (Fig 6).

The study [66] supports the findings of previous studies [62, 63] with no change in the MEP amplitude despite strength increases. However, the significance of this study is two-fold: 1) this is the first study to measure and report SP data with a strength training study; and 2) SP duration was significantly reduced in the trained group and correlated with the observed increase in strength. These findings demonstrate that in this study using a hand muscle, strength training has positively altered the effectivenes of the cortical inhibitory circuits that project onto the FDI. The reasons for this are unclear; however, with the hypothesis that strength training is a form of skill training [46, 60, 61], the repetitive nature of the strength training regime may have induced a task-dependant neural adaptation in corticospinal output [23, 38].

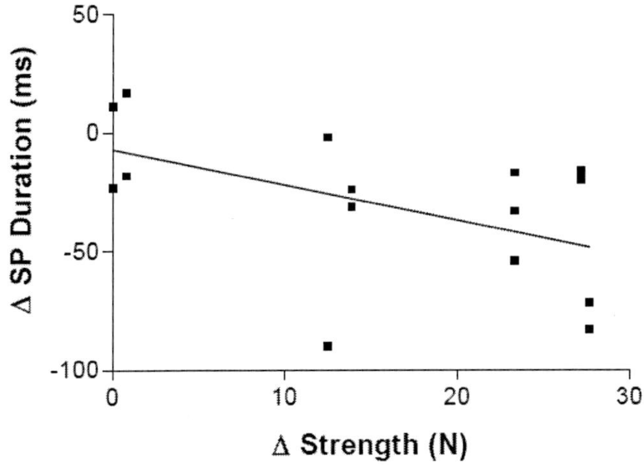

Figure 6. The relationship between changes (as represented by delta [△]) in strength of the right FDI and pooled SP duration of the strength trained group (r=-0.51, p=0.05) [66].

The study did not support the findings of Griffen and Cafarelli [64], and Beck et al [65]. However, it should be noted that both of these studies [64, 65] investigated strength training involving the tibialis anterior, reporting increased MEP amplitude. These contrasting findings may be explained through task orientated differences in muscles used predominately for fine motor tasks (such as the hand) versus muscles used for gross movements with a strength component (such as the leg). Therefore, in order to explore this further, the second study [67] and third studies [68] conducted investigated corticospinal excitability and inhibition following four weeks of heavy load strength training of the elbow flexor muscles.

TMS evoked MEPs were recorded from the right biceps brachii (BB) muscle from 24 individuals (26.8 ± 7.3 years; training group n=13, control group n=11), novice to strength training, before and after four weeks of progressive overload strength training at 80% of one-repetition maximum (1RM). Participants' completed 12 supervised strength training sessions that involved 4 sets of 8 repetitions of a standard bicep curl exercise. Previous research has demonstrated that slow velocity strength training is associated with a greater level of neural adaptation compared to high velocity strength training alone and it is thought such adaptations may be mediated by peripheral feedback mechanisms [69, 70], therefore, each bicep curl repetition was performed with a 3 s concentric (flexion) phase and 4 s eccentric (extension) phase.

Measures included measurement of 1RM strength [71], upper arm circumference [71], sEMG and stimulus-response (SR) curves [26]. SR curves (Fig 7) were applied, before and after the four week training program, by increasing the stimulator output from 30% (of stimulator output) increasing in 5% steps until the saturation of the MEP (MEP_{max}). At each stimulus intensity, 10 stimuli were delivered whilst the participant was maintaining a 10% of MVC sEMG tonic contraction.

SR curves were calculated by plotting the stimulus intensity against MEP amplitude, and the data was fitted with a three parameter sigmoid equation:

$$MEP(s) = \frac{MEP_{MAX}}{1 + e^{m(S50-s)}}$$

Where *s* is stimulus intensity, *m* is the estimated slope, *S50* is the estimated peak slope, and MEP_{max} is the measured maximum the participant's MEP amplitude reached in a given trial. A non-linear data fit iterative model to each participant's data using SPSS (V17.0) was applied. This procedure estimated the values for *m* and *S50* and provided a measure of the curves fit to the data.

Table 1 illustrates pre and post training strength and TMS data between groups. Strength training resulted in a 28% increase (p=0.001) in 1RM strength (with no change in the bicep brachii girth). No differences in strength or muscle girth were observed in the control group.

Figure 7 shows training group mean MEP SR curves pre (Fig 7a) and post (Fig 7b) training. No significant differences for the percentage of stimulator output at AMT within and between groups pre- (p=0.31) and post-training (p=0.83) were observed (Table 1). Similarly there were no significant differences in pre-training mean MEP amplitude at all stimulus intensities at and above AMT between the groups ($p = 0.16$). However, following training, there was a significant increase in mean MEP amplitude at AMT in the trained group ($p = 0.05$; Fig 7ii) and at stimulus intensities at 20% above (p=0.05) and MEP_{max} (p=0.02; Fig 7ii) which was not observed in the control group (Table 1). The increased MEP amplitudes at 20% and MEP_{max} did not significantly affect the estimated slope (*m*; p=0.36) or estimated peak slope (*S50*; p=0.61) of the curve (Table 1).

Contrary to our previous study [66] SP remained unchanged in both groups, pre and post training. Therefore the findings in this study, supporting previous investigations [64, 65], demonstrate that in a gross muscle (such as the BB) corticospinal excitability has increased in response to four weeks of repeated bouts of heavy load strength training.

Table 1. Mean data (± SD) for percentage of stimulator output at aMT (%), MEP amplitude at AMT (mV), 20% above aMT (mV), maximum MEP_{max} (mV), SP duration (msec) at 20% above aMT (mV) and at MEP_{max} (ms), prior to and following the four week strength training intervention for the control and trained groups left M1. Asterisk indicates statistical significance ($p < 0.05$) [67]

	Strength (1RM)		Stimulator Output at aMT (%)		aMT amplitude (mV)		MEP Amplitude (mV) @ 20% above AMT		Max MEP (mV)		SP Duration (ms) at 20% above AMT		SP Duration (ms) at Max MEP (Mmax)	
	Pre	Post	Pre	Post	Pre	Post	Pre	Post	Pre	Post	Pre	Post	Pre	Post
Control	13.33 ± 4.26	13.28± 4.33	49.37± 6.70	45.62± 7.70	1.04± 0.72	0.78± 0.19	2.87± 1.42	2.76± 0.93	3.35± 1.81	3.39 1.34	96.60± 18.20	99.65± 12.80	115.75± 12.94	114.23± 15.05
Trained	11.50± 4.52	14.77± 5.22*	50.0± 10.40	49.5 ± 9.60	0.82± 0.28	1.26± 0.51*	2.45± 0.92	3.26± 1.19 *	2.81± 0.96	3.89± 1.09 *	107.93± 23.90	104.91± 18.86	112.07± 17.36	107.86± 22.41

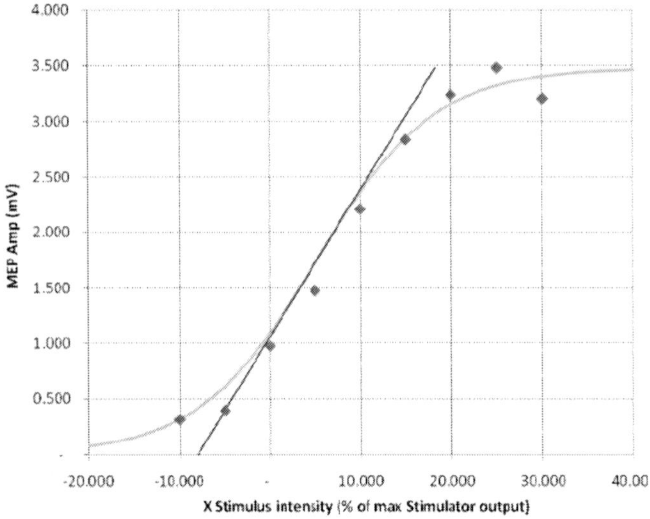

a

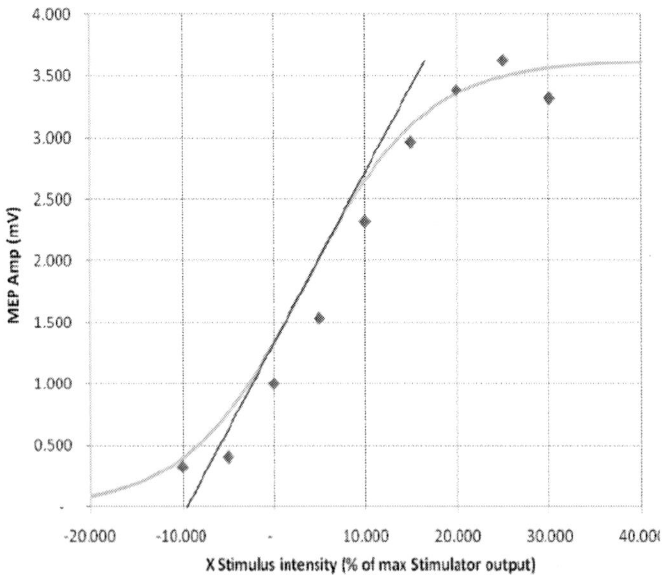

b

Figure 7a and b. Calculated and fitted sigmoid curves over collected from SR curves (10% below individual's threshold [-] to 30% above threshold) pre (a) and post (b) intervention in the training group. Asterisk indicated significant difference in calculated curve fit at T, ($p<0.05$) [68].

From the limited data to date, it is reasonable to suggest that neural adaptations underpin short-term strength increases following training of a muscle. Moreover the adaptations that occur, despite having commonalities with skill training adaptations, may differ depending on the muscle used for training. Given that intrinsic hand muscles are used primarily for fine skilled tasks, the muscle tested (FDI) and movement protocol used in the first study (simple abduction movement) may not have been satisfactorily challenging the corticospinal pathway to reflect changes in MEP amplitude [50, 51] despite maximal isometric activation and an increase in strength. However, using a heavy load training protocol in larger gross muscles, primarily used for strength tasks, resulted in increased MEP amplitudes. The corticospinal excitability increases shown in the second study are likely to be explained by changes in cortical synapse number and/or synaptic strength [72, 73] responding to the repetitive nature of the training using a muscle ideally suited to high force production. Despite employing a relatively simple movement (elbow flexion and extension), the requirement of participants' to control the exercise inherently created a skilled element which may have also contributed to increased corticospinal excitability using similar physiological processes originating in the cerebral cortex [46, 59].

Strength-Training and the Cross-Transfer of Strength

The final study to be presented in this chapter presents recent research [68] investigating the neural mechanisms underpinning cross-education (also known as bilateral transfer) training. Initially described in 1894 by Scripture and colleagues [74], whereby unilateral motor training of one limb improves motor task performance of the contralateral limb, there is good evidence to support cross-education in strength training of upper and lower limbs showing increases in strength of the untrained limb, in the absence of hypertrophy [46, 59].

Neurophysiological mechanisms underpinning cross-education have been suggested [59], and demonstrated with evidence stemming from motor skill acquisition [75- 78] and strength training literature [70, 79-82]. Some authors have also employed unfamiliar movement training demonstrating cross-education strength. For example, Farthing et al [83] had participants' strength train forearm muscles using a relatively unfamiliar ulna deviation movement showing improvements in the untrained arm; concluding that neural adaptations arose as a result from strength but also efficiency in movement suggesting similar neural pathways adapt and respond following strength training *and* skill acquisition [46]. However, to the best of our knowledge, currently no data is available on corticospinal responses to the untrained limb following cross-education training using heavy load (80% of 1RM) unilateral isotonic strength training of the forearm flexor muscles.

This study used a similar between-groups and training protocol design to our previous strength training study presented earlier in the chapter [66]. The trained group (6 males, 20.3 ± 3.4 years and 7 females, 24.5 ± 3.0 years) completed four weeks of supervised unilateral strength training (ULS) of the right BB (4 sets of 8 repetitions, with controlled repetition speed of 3 s concentric/4 s eccentric) with the control group (6 males, 27.6 ± 7.9 years and 5 females, 29 ± 6.2 years) not participating in any training, only attending the pre and post testing sessions.

TMS evoked MEPs were recorded via sEMG from the left BB (right M1) whilst participants held a low level tonic contraction of 10% of MVC sEMG. Pre- and post-training SR curves, maximal strength (in both arms), upper arm girths, sEMG activity, latency, MEP amplitude and SP duration were applied and quantified using methods previously described in chapter 1.

For both groups there were no changes in left BB girth, pre and post training (p=0.40). Unilateral strength training resulted in 28% increase in 1RM right elbow flexion strength, in the trained group, resulting in an associated 19.2% increase in strength in the untrained arm (r=0.62, p=0.02; Fig 8). No differences pre- and post-training, and between groups, were observed for latency and SP duration. Comparison of calculated SR curves showed, for the trained group, 33% increase at 20% above AMT (p=0.03) and a 26.5% increase at MEP_{max} (p=0.01).

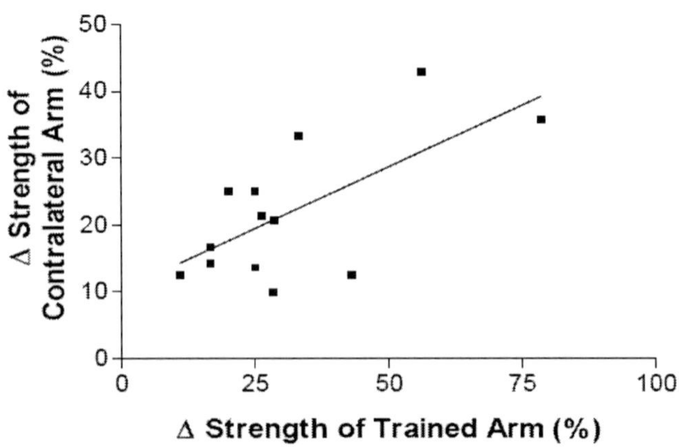

Figure 8. Association of strength changes (expressed as a percentage of pre-training strength and represented by delta [△]) between the elbow flexors of the trained and contralateral untrained limb in the trained group after four-weeks of heavy load controlled unilateral strength training (r = 0.67; p=0 .05) [68].

The findings of this study extend on previous work demonstrating neurophysiological mechanisms underpinning the cross-education of strength [83]. There are two evidence-based explanations to currently explain the mechanisms of cross-education. These include ipsilateral corticospinal projections and motor irradiation. Anatomically, it has been shown that 10% [84, 85] to 30% [86] of pyramidal tract neurons do not decussate providing ipsilateral corticospinal projections. Paired-pulse TMS studies [23] have recently demonstrated increased MEP amplitudes in ipsilateral corticospinal projections following wrist flexion of increasing force further supporting the contribution of ipsilateral corticospinal pathways. Our study did not measure ipsilateral MEPs, however, the findings of increased excitability in the contralateral (right) M1 support the motor irradiation theory [46, 59, 87], that cortical activity during strong unilateral contractions diffuse from the active M1 to the "inactive" M1 giving rise to bilateral activation of both motor cortices. Mountcastle [88] has proposed this occurs through interhemispheric pathways via cortico-cortical cells within layer II and III of the M1 forming a broad, intrinsic horizontal projection system. Neuro-imaging and TMS studies have shown mechanisms whereby unilateral motor activity is associated with bilateral activation of both the left and right M1 [23, 87, 89, 90] via increased excitability of existing intrinsic horizontal pathways within the M1.

Similar to our previous strength training studies [66, 67], the repeated strong and controlled movement tasks may have also induced a motor learning effect. A general consensus exists in the literature that cross-education of strength might be similar to cross-education of motor skill acquisition[46, 59, 62]. Carroll et al. [62] has put forward that strength training is a form of motor learning, in the sense that participants are required to learn to produce muscle recruitment patterns associated with optimal performance of the task. Other authors concur that short-term increases in strength stem from improved coordination [60, 61, 91, 92]. Moreover, Farthing and Chilibek [80] have affirmed that skill learning does not induce muscle hypertrophy but still contributes to gains in strength. As proposed by Parlow and Kinsbourne [77], the cross-education model suggests that motor task or skill memory engrams are stored in both hemispheres following unilateral skill acquisition, and the findings from recent studies, described above, suggest that it is plausible that this also occurs with unilateral strength training.

CONCLUSION

This text has described several of our studies investigating the mechanisms of neural adaptations following skill and strength training. For both acute skill [50, 51], long term skill [43] and strength studies [66-68], neural adaptations may be attributed to a number of proposed mechanisms: rapid responses to precision movements in corticospinal excitability include changes in cortical synaptic strength [93, 94]; unmasking of pre-existing connections in the M1 [96] where older neural pathways, potentially made redundant due to newer pathways taking over, reactivate; or the change in balance between excitatory or inhibitory inputs from presynaptic neurons thereby altering the excitability or inhibition of existing neural connections [96]. A suggestion still open to conjecture [97] is the activation of existing or "silent" synapses defined as a connection between synapses but presynaptic neurotransmitter release does not result in graded or action potenials in postsynaptic neurons [98]. The activation of these "silent" synapses has been shown experimentally [99] and in animal models [100], however, there is little evidence of the existence of silent synapses in the mature human nervous system. Although, as proposed by Rioult-Pedotti and Donoghue [97], the activation of silent synapses is a theoretically plausible component underpinning neuroplasticity.

Longer term neuroplastic changes, as presented in the badminton study [43] can be attributed to the mechanisms of long term potentiation (LTP) or long term depression or inhibition (LTD or LTI) [101, 102]. LTP refers to a persistent increase in synaptic efficacy between presynaptic and postsynaptic neurons and has been suggested as a mechanism to consolidate learning. Alternatively, LTD increases the inhibition between neurones actively altering the threshold for the post synaptic neurone to generate an action potential. LTP has been demonstrated to be involved in the learning as well as the retention of motor skills [103, 104] as well as long term expert motor performance [43].

Motor learning and memory of skills has also been attributed to new synapses (synaptogenesis) or remodelling of existing synapses (synaptic remodelling) underpinning LTP. Evidence of increased synapses per neuron following a period of motor skill learning have been shown in M1 [105] and the cerebellum [106, 107]. However, contradictory evidence has been presented with a number of studies showing evidence for increased synapse numbers [108, 109] or no change [109, 110] following learning or LTP induction. For further reading on LTP and synapto-genesis the reader is directed to review by Geinisman [111].

To date, the data collected and presented in this text has been on healthy, able individuals; however, neuroplasticity's real value lies in benefiting those with dysfunction or disability, such as those with neurological conditions. It is recognised that neuroplasticity occurs following skill training, but research focus is now to investigate the benefits of using exercise, particularly strength training in those with neurological conditions. Fox et al [113] in discussing the benefits of exercise augmenting neuroplasticity, particularly in relation to Parkinson's disease but quite suitable to a number of neurological conditions, suggest five principles underpinning this mechanism: (1) intensive exercise maximizes synaptic plasticity; (2) complex tasks promote adaptation; (3) tasks that are rewarding increase dopamine levels, promoting learning/relearning; (4) dopaminergic neurons are highly responsive to exercise, but also to inactivity; and (5) where exercise is introduced at an earlier stage of the disease, progression hypothetically may be slowed. There is good evidence that functional outcomes are achieved using exercise as therapy [114, 115], and attributing improvements to neuroplasticity. Future research in our laboratory will be aiming to investigate the mechanisms underpinning studies demonstrating benefits of exercise to those with neurological conditions.

ACKNOWLEDGMENTS

We are only beginning our journey into looking at neural adaptations with strength training, but have a number of colleagues to thank for helping us to this point. We would like to thank Dr Mark Stokes for his mathematical assistance in calculating the stimulus-response curves; Mr Troy Castrium and Mr Scott Hunter for their assistance with the strength training projects, and Professor Gary Thickbroom for his assistance with the skill acquisition studies. Finally we are indebted to the support and vision by Professors John Carlson, David Crawford and David Cameron-Smith for assisting us in setting up our labs and encouraging us to pursue our passion in the discipline of exercise neuroscience.

References

[1] Thickbroom, G. W., & Mastaglia F. L. (2009) Plasticity in neurological disorders and challenges for noninvasive brain stimulation (NBS). *Journal of Neuroengineering and Rehabilitation* [Online serial], 6: 4.

[2] Fuhr, P., Cohen, L. G., Dang, N., Findlay, T. W., Haghighi, S., Oro, J., & Hallett M. (1992) Physiological analysis of motor reorganization following lower limb amputation. *Electroencephalography and Clinical neurophysiology 85:* 53-60.

[3] Cohen, L. G., Bandinelli, S., Findley, T. W., & Hallett M. (1991) Motor reorganization after upper limb amputation in man. *Brain 114:* 615-627.

[4] Brasil-Neto, J. P., Cohen, L. G., Pasual-Leone, A., Jabir, F. K., Wall, R. T., & Hallett, M. (1992) Rapid reversible modulation of human motor outputs after transient deafferentation of the forearm: A study with transcranial magnetic stimulation. *Neurology 42:* 1302-1306.

[5] Byrnes, M. L., Thickbroom, G. W., Phillips, B. A., Wilson, S. A., & Mastaglia, F. L. (1999) Physiological studies of the corticomotor projection to the hand after subcortical stroke. *Clinical Neurophysiology 110:* 487-498.

[6] Byrnes, M. L., Thickbroom, G. W., Wilson, S. A., Shipman, J. M., Stell, R., & Mastaglia, F.L. (1998) The corticomotor representation of upper limb muscles in writer's cramp and changes following botulinum toxin injection. *Brain 121:* 977-988.

[7] Thickbroom, G. W., Byrnes, M. L., Walters, S., Stell, R., & Mastaglia, F. L. (2006) Motor cortex reorganisation in Parkinson's disease. *Journal of Clinical Neuroscience 13*: 639-642.

[8] Lee, M., Reddy, H., Johansen-Berg, H., Pendlebury, S., Jenkinson, M., Smith, S. et al (2000) The motor cortex shows adaptive functional changes to brain injury from multiple sclerosis. *Annals of Neurology 47:* 606-613.

[9] Barker, A. T., Jalinous, R., & Freeston, I. L. (1985) Non-invasive magnetic stimulation of human motor cortex. *Lancet 2:* 1106-1107.

[10] Wassermann E. M. (2002) Safety and side-effects of transcranial magnetic stimulation and repetitive transcranial magnetic stimulation. In: A. P. Pascual-Leone, N. J. Davey, J. C. Rothwell, E. M. Wasserman, & B. K. Puri (Eds.) *Handbook of Transcranial Magnetic Stimulation* (pp. 39-49). New York: Oxford University Press.

[11] Gilbert, D. L., Garvey, M. A., Bansal, A. S., Lipps T, Zhang J, & Wassermann EM (2004). Should transcranial magnetic stimulation research in children be considered minimal risk? *Clinical Neurophysiology 115:* 1730-1739.

[12] Quintana, H. (2005) Transcranial magnetic stimulation in persons younger than the age of 18. *Journal of Electroconvulsive Therapy, 21:* 88-95.

[13] Hallett, M. (2000) Transcranial magnetic stimulation and the human brain. *Nature 406:* 147-150.

[14] Hallett, M. (2007) Transcranial Magnetic Stimulation: A Primer. *Neuron 55:* 187-199.

[15] Kidgell, D. J., & Pearce, A. J. (2009) Neural adaptations following cross education strength training. *Journal of Science and Medicine in Sport 12:* 52-53.

[16] Hess, C. W., Mills, K. R., & Murrary, N. M. F. (1987). Reponses in small hand muscles from magnetic stimulation of the human brain. *Journal of Physiology, 388*: 397-419.

[17] Mills, K. R., & Murray, N. M. F. (1986). Corticospinal tract conduction time in multiple sclerosis. *Annual of Neurology, 18:* 601-605.

[18] Rossini, P. M., Barker, A. T., Berardelli, A., Caramia, M. D., Caruso, G., Cracco R. Q., et al (1994) Non-invasive electrical and magnetic stimulation of the brain, spinal cord and roots: basic principles and procedures for routine clinical application. Report of an IFCN committee. *Electroencephalography and Clinical Neurophysiology 91:* 79-92.

[19] Rosler, K. M. (2001) Transcranial magnetic brain stimulation: a tool to investigate central motor pathways. *News in Physiological Science 16:* 297-302

[20] Wassermann, E. M. (2005) Individual differences in the response to transcranial magnetic stimulation. In: M. Hallett, S. Chokroverty (eds) Magnetic stimulation in clinical neurophysiology (pp. 303-310). Philadelphia: Elsevier.

[21] Kamen, G. (2004) Reliability of motor-evoked potentials during resting and active contraction conditions. *Medicine and Science in Sports and Exercise 36:* 1574-1579.

[22] van Hedel, H., Murer, C., Dietz, V., & Curt, A. (2007) The amplitude of lower leg motor evoked potentials is a reliable measure when controlled for torque and motor task. *Journal of Neurology 254:* 1089-1098

[23] Perez, M.A., & Cohen, L.G. (2008) Mechanisms underlying functional changes in the primary motor cortex ipsilateral to an active hand. *Journal of Neuroscience 28:* 5631-5640

[24] Pearce, A.J. (2000) Physiological studies in the human corticomotor system associated with dynamic and static movement. PhD thesis, University of Western Australia.

[25] Cantello, R., Gianelli, M., Civardi, C., & Mutani, R. (1992). Magnetic brain stimulation:The silent period after the motor evoked potential. *Neurology, 42:* 1951-1959.

[26] Wilson, S. A., Lockwood, R. J., Thickbroom, G. W., & Mastaglia, F. L. (1993). The muscle silent period following transcranial magnetic cortical stimulation. *Journal of the Neurological Sciences, 114*: 216-222.

[27] Chen, R., Lozano, A. M., & Ashby, P. (1999). Mechanism of the silent period following transcranial magnetic stimulation Evidence from epidural recordings. *Experimental Brain Research 128*: 539-542.

[28] Werhahn, K. J., Kunesch, E., Noachtar, S., Benecke, R., & Classen, J. (1999). Differential effects on motorcortical inhibition induced by blockade of GABA uptake in humans. *Journal of Physiology 517:* 591-597

[29] Werhahn KJ, Behrang-Nia M, Bott MC, & Klimpe S (2007) Does the Recruitment of Excitation and Inhibition in the Motor Cortex Differ? *Journal of Clinical Neurophysiology 24:* 419-423.

[30] Werhahn, K. J., Classen, J. & Benecke, R. (1995). The silent period induced by transcranial magnetic stimulation in muscles supplied by cranial nerves: normal data and changes in patients. *Journal of Neurology Neurosurgery and Psychiatry 59:* 586-96.

[31] Davey, N.J., Romaiguere, P., Maskill, D.W., & Ellaway, P.H. (1994) Suppression of voluntary motor activity revealed using transcranial magnetic stimulation of the motor cortex in man. *Journal of Physiology 477:* 223-235

[32] Hess, A., Kunesch, E., Classen, J., Hoeppner, J., Stefan, K., & Benecke, R. (1999). Task-dependant modulation of inhibitory actions within the primary motor cortex. *Experimental Brain Research, 124:* 321-330.

[33] Haug, B. A., Schonle, P. W., Knobloch, C., & Kohne, M. (1992). Silent period measurement revives as a valuable diagnostic tool with transcranial magnetic stimulation. *Electroencephalography and Clinical Neurophysiology, 85:* 158-160.

[34] Classen, J., & Benecke, R. (1995). Inhibitory phenomena in individual motor units induced by transcranial magnetic stimulation. *Electroencephalography and clinical Neurophysiology, 97:* 264-274.

[35] Classen, J., Schnitzler, A., Binkofski, F., Werhahn, K. J., Kim, Y.-S., Kessler, K. R., et al. (1997). The motor syndrome associated with exaggerated inhibition within the primary motor cortex of patients with hemiparetic stroke. *Brain, 120:* 605-619.

[36] Pascual-Leone, A. P., Davey, N. J., Rothwell, J. C., Wasserman, E. M. & Puri B. K. *Handbook of Transcranial Magnetic Stimulation.* New York: Oxford University Press.

[37] Boniface, S., & Siemann, U. (2003).Plasticity in the Human Nervous System. Cambridge: Cambridge University Press.

[38] Pascaul-Leone, A., Dang, N., Cohen, L. G., Brasil-Neto, J.P., Cammarota, A., & Hallett, M. (1995) Modulation of muscle responses evoked by transcrannial magnetic stimulation during the acquisition of new fine motor skills. *Journal of Neurophysiology 74:* 1037-1043

[39] Pascual-Leone, A. (1996) Reorganisation of cortical motor outputs in theacquisition of new motor skills. In: J. Kimura, H. Shibasaki (Eds) *Xth International Congress of EMG and Clinical Neurophysiology* (pp. 304-308). Elsevier, Kyoto.

[40] Rothwell, J. C. (1994). *Control of Voluntary Human Movement.* London, Chapman & Hall.

[41] Bohning, D. E., Shasri, A., McConnell, K. A., Nahas, Z., Lorderbaum, J. P., Roberts, D. R. et al (1999) A combined TMS/fMRI study of intensity-dependent TMS over motor cortex. *Biological Psychiatry 45:* 385-394.

[42] Kuhtz-Buschbeck, J.P., Mahnkopf, C., Holzknecht, C., Siebner, H., Ulmer, S., & Jansen, O. (2003) Effector-independent representation of simple and complex imagined finger movements: a combined fMRI and TMS study. *European Journal of Neuroscience 18:* 3375-3387.

[43] Pearce, A. J., Thickbroom, G. W., Byrnes, M. L., & Mastaglia, F. L. (2000). The corticomotor representation of elite racquet sport athletes. *Experimental Brain Research, 130:* 238-243

[44] Thickbroom, G. W., & Mastaglia, F. L. (1998). Mapping studies. In A. Pascual-Leone, N. J. Davey, J. C. Rothwell, E. M. Wassermann, & B. K. Puri (Eds.), *Handbook of Magnetic Stimulation* (pp. 127-140) New York: Oxford University Press.

[45] Semmler, J. G., & Enoka, R. M. (2000) Neural contributions to changes in muscle strength. In: Zatsiorski V (Ed) *Biomechanics in Sport: Performance Enhancement and Injury Prevention* (pp 3-20). London: Blackwell Science.

[46] Farthing, J. P. (2009) Cross-Education of Strength Depends on Limb Dominance: Implications for Theory and Application. *Exercise and Sport Sciences Reviews 37:* 179-187

[47] Datta, A. K., Harrison, L. M., & Stephens, J. A. (1989). Task-dependant changes in the size of response to magnetic brain stimulation in human first dorsal interosseous muscle. *Journal of Physiology 418:* 13-23.

[48] Flament, D., Goldsmith, P., Buckley, C. J., & Lemon, R. N. (1993). Task dependance of responses in first dorsal interosseous muscle to magnetic brain stimulation in man. *Journal of Physiology 464:* 361-378.

[49] Schieppati, M., Trompetto C., & Abbruzzese G. (1996) Selective facilitation of responses to cortical stimulation of proximal and distal arm muscles by precision tasks in man. *Journal of Physiology 491:* 551-562

[50] Pearce, A.J., & Kidgell, D. J. (2009) Corticomotor excitability during precision motor tasks. *Journal of Science and Medicine in Sport 12:* 280-283.

[51] Pearce, A.J, & Kidgell, D.J. (2010) Comparison of corticomotor excitability during visuomotor dynamic and static tasks. *Journal of Science and Medicine in Sport 13:* 167-171.

[52] Karni, A., Meyer, G., Jezzard, P., Adams, M.M., Turner, R., & Ungerlelder, L. G. (1995) Functional MRI evidence for adult motor cortex plasticity during motor skill learning. *Nature 377:* 155-158

[53] Wang, Y., Sereno, J.A., Jongman, A., & Hirsch, J. (2003) fMRI evidence for cortical modification during learning of Mandarin lexical tone. *Journal of Cognitive Neuroscience 15:* 1019-1027

[54] Ericsson, K.A., Krampe, R.T., & Tesch-Römer, C. (1993) The role of deliberate practice. *Psychological Review 100:* 363-406

[55] Elbert ,T., Pantev, C., Wienbruch, C., Rockstroh, B., & Taub, E. (1995) Increased cortical representation of the fingers of the left hand in string players. *Science 270:* 305-307.

[56] Bryden, M.P. (1977) Measuring handedness with questionnaires *Neuropsychologica 15:* 617-624.

[57] Sale, D.G. (1988) Neural adaptation to resistance training. *Medicine and Science in Sports and Exercise 20:* s135-s145.

[58] Folland, J. P., & Williams, A. G. (2007). The adaptations to strength training : morphological and neurological contributions to increased strength. *Sports Medicine 37:* 145-168.

[59] Zhou, S. (2000). Chronic neural adaptations to unilateral exercise: mechanisms of cross education. *Exercise and Sports Science Reviews 28:* 177-184.

[60] Faigenbaum, A.D., Loud, R.L., O'Connell, J., Glover, S., O'Connell, J. & Westcott, W.L. (2001) Effects of different resistance training protocols on

upper-body strength and endurance development in children. *Journal of Strength Conditioning Research, 15:* 459-465.

[61] Faigenbaum, A.D., Zaichkowsky, L.D., Wescott, W.L., Micheli, L., & Fehlandt, A.F. (1993). The effects of twice a week strength training program on children. *Paediatric Exercise Science, 5:* 339-346.

[62] Carroll, T. J., Riek, S., & Carson, R. G. (2002). The sites of neural adaptation induced by resistance training in humans. *Journal of Physiology 544:* 641-652.

[63] Jensen, J. L., Marstrand, P. C., & Nielsen, J. B. (2005). Motor skill training and strength training are associated with different plastic changes in the central nervous system. *Journal of Applied Physiology 99:* 1558-1568.

[64] Griffin, L., & Cafarelli, E. (2007). Transcranial magnetic stimulation during resistance training of the tibialis anterior muscle. *Journal of Electromyography and Kinesiology 17:* 446-452.

[65] Beck, S., Taube, W., Gruber, M., Amtage, F., Gollhofer, A., & Schubert, M. (2007). Task-specific changes in motor evoked potentials of lower limb muscles after different training interventions. *Brain Research 1179*: 51-60.

[66] Kidgell, D. J., & Pearce, A. J. (In Press). Corticospinal properties and force steadiness following short-term strength training of an intrinsic hand muscle. *Human Movement Science.*

[67] Kidgell, D. J., Stokes, M.A., Castrium, T., & Pearce, A.J. (In Press). Neurophysiological responses following short-term strength training of the biceps brachii muscle. *Journal of Strength and Conditioning.*

[68] Kidgell, D. J., Stokes, M. A., Pearce, A. J. (In Press). Strength training of one limb increases corticomotor excitability projecting to the contralateral homologous limb. *Motor Control.*

[69] Hortobágyi, T., Hill, J. P., Houmard, J. A., Fraser, D. D. Lambert N. J. & Isreal R. G. (1996). Adaptive responses to muscle lengthening and shortening in humans. *Journal of Applied Physiology 80*: 765-772.

[70] Hortobágyi, T., Lambert, N. J., & Hill, J. P. (1997). Greater cross education following training with muscle lengthening than shortening. *Medicine and Science in Sports and Exercise 29:* 107-112.

[71] Munn, J., Herbert, R. D., Hancock, M. J., & Gandevia, S. C. (2005). Resistance training for strength: effect of number of sets and contraction speed. *Medicine and Science in Sports and Exercise 37:* 1622-1626.

[72] Chen, R., Yaseen, Z. Cohen, L. G., & Hallett, M.. (1998). Time course of corticospinal excitability in reaction time and self-paced movements. *Annals of Neurology 44:* 317 - 325.

[73] Ridding, M. C., & J. C. Rothwell (1997). Stimulus/response curves as a method of measuring motor cortical excitability in man. *Electroencephalogry and Clinical Neurophysiology 105:* 340-344.

[74] Scripture, E. W., T. L. Smith, Brown, E.M. (1894). On the education of muscular control and power. *Studies Yale Psychology Laboratory 2:* 114-119.

[75] Imamizu H., & Shimojo S. (1995). The locus of visual-motor learning at the task or manipulator level: Implications from intermanual transfer. Journal of *Experimental Psychology and Human Perceptual Performance. 21:*719-733.

[76] Parlow S.E., & Kinsbourne M. (1989). Asymmetrical transfer of training between hands: Implications for interhemispheric communication in normal brain. *Brain Cognition. 11:* 98-113.

[77] Stoddard J., & Vaid J (1996). Asymmetries in intermanual transfer of maze learning in right- and left-handed adults. *Neuropsychologia 34:* 605-608.

[78] Katrin, S., Lüders, E., Jäncke, L. (2002). Intermanual Transfer in a Simple Motor Task. *Cortex 38:* 805-815.

[79] Teixeira, L. A, & Caminha L. Q. (2003). Intermanual transfer of force control is modulated by asymmetry of muscular strength. *Experimental Brain Research 149:* 312-319.

[80] Farthing J.P., & Chilibeck, P.D. (2003). The effects of eccentric training at different velocities on cross-education. *European Journal of. Applied Physiology 89:*570-577.

[81] Farthing, J.P., Chilibeck, P.D., & Binsted, G. (2005) Cross-dducation of arm muscular strength Is unidirectional in right-handed Individuals. *Medicine & Science in Sports & Exercise 37:* 1594-1600

[82] Lee, M., Gandevia, S. C., & Carroll, T. J. (2009). Unilateral strength training increases voluntary activation of the opposite untrained limb. *Clinical Neurophysiology* 120: 802-808.

[83] Farthing J. P., Borowsky R., Chilibeck P.D., Binsted, G., & Sarty, G. (2007) Neuro-physiological adaptations associated with cross-education of strength. *Brain Topography 20:* 77-88.

[84] Nyberg-Hansen, R., & Rinvik, E. (1963). Some comments on the pyramidal tract, with special reference to its individual variations in man. *Acta Neurologica Scandinavia 39:* 1-30.

[85] Carpenter, M. B. *Core text of neuroanatomy*. Baltimore: Williams & Wilkins. 1985.

[86] Nathan, P. W., Smith, M. C., & Deacon, P. (1990). The corticospinal tracts in man. Course and location of fibres at different segmental levels (Pt 2). *Brain 113:* 303-324.

[87] Todor, J. I., & Lazarus, J. A. (1986). Exertion level and the intensity of associated movements. *Developmental Medicine and Child Neurology 28*: 205-212.

[88] Mountcastle, V. B. (1997). The columnar organization of the neocortex. *Brain 120:* 701-722.

[89] Hortobágyi, T., Taylor, J. L., Petersen, N. T., Russell, G., & Gandevia, S. C. (2003). Changes in segmental and motor cortical output with contralateral muscle contractions and altered sensory inputs in humans. *Journal of Neurophysioly 90*: 2451-2459.

[90] Hortobágyi, T. (2005). Cross education and the human central nervous system. *IEEE Engineering and Medical Biological Magazine 24*: 22-28.

[91] Enoka, R. M. (1997). Neural adaptations with chronic physical activity. *Journal of Biomechanics 30:* 447-455.

[92] Olafsdottir, H. B., Zatsiorsky, V. M., & Latash, M. L. (2008). The effects of strength training on finger strength and hand dexterity in healthy elderly individuals. *Journal of Applied Physiology 105:* 1166-1178.

[93] Jones, T. A. (1999). Multiple synapse formation in the motor cortex opposite unilateral sensorimotor cortex lesions in adult rats. *Journal of Compartive Neurology 414*: 57-66.

[94] Muellbacher, W., Ziemann, U. , Boroojerdi, B., Cohen, L. G., & Hallett, M. (2001). Role of the human motor cortex in rapid motor learning. *Experimental Brain Research 136*: 431-438.

[95] Huntley, G. W. (1997). Correlations between patterns of horizontal connectivity and the extent of short-term representational plasticity in rat motor cortex. *Cerebral Cortex 7:*143-156.

[96] Jacobs, K.M., & Donoghue, J.P. (1991). Reshaping the cortical motor map by unmasking latent intracortical connection. *Science 251:* 944-947.

[97] Rioult-Pedotti, M-S., & Donoghue, J.P. (2003). The nature and mechanisms of plasticity. In: S. Boniface, & U. Ziemann U (Eds) *Plasticity in the human nervous system: Investigations with transcranial magnetic stimulation* (pp 1-25). Cambridge: Cambridge University Press.

[98] Liao, D.N., Hessler, A., & Malinow, R. (1995). Activation of postsynaptically silent synapses during pairing-induced LTP in CA1 region of hippocampal slice. *Nature 375:* 400-404.

[99] Liao, D. N., Zhang, X., O'Brien, R., Ehlers, M. D., & Huganir, R. L. (1999). Regulation of morphological postsynaptic silent synapses in developing hippocampal neurons. *Nature Neuroscience 2:* 37-43.

[100] Atwood, H.L., & Wojitowicz, J.M. (1999). Silent synapses in neural plasticity: current evidence. *Learning and Memory 6:* 542-571.

[101] Bliss, T.V.P., & Lomo, T. (1973). Long-lasting potentiation of synaptic transmission in the dentate area of the anesthetised rabbit following stimulation of the perforant path. *Journal of Physiology 232:* 331-356.

[102] Martin, S.J., Grimwood, P.D., & Morris, R.G.M. (2000) Synaptic plasticity and memory: an evaluation of the hypothesis. *Annual Review of Neurosicence 23:* 649-711.

[103] Rioult-Pedotti, M-S., Friedman, D., & Donoghue, J.P. (2000). Learning-induced LTP in neocortex. *Science 290:* 533-536.

[104] Rioult-Pedotti, M-S., & Donoghue, J.P. (2002). Learning, retention and persistent strengthening of cortical synapses. *Society of Neuroscience 32:* 713.

[105] Kleim, J.A., Lussing, E., Schwarz, E.R., Comery, T. A., & Greenough, W. T. (1996) Synaptogenesis and FOS expression in the motor cortex of adult rat after motor skill learning. *Journal of Neuroscience 16:* 4529-4535.

[106] Kleim, J.A., Vij, K., Ballard, D.H., & Greenough, W. T. (1997) Learning dependent synaptic modifications in the cerebellar cortex of the adult rat persist at least four weeks. *Journal of Neuroscience 17:* 717-721.

[107] Kleim, J.A., Barbay, S., & Nudo, R.J. (1998). Functional reorganisation of the rat motor cortex following motor skill learning. *Journal of Neurophysiology 80:* 3321-3325.

[108] Engert, F., Bonhoeffer, T. (1999). Dendritic spine changes associated with hippocampal lonterm synaptic plasticity. *Nature 399:* 66-70.

[109] Toni, B., Buchs, P-A., Nikonenko, I., Bron, C. R., & Muller, D. (1999). LTP promotes formation of multiple spin synapses between a single axon terminal and a dendrite. *Nature 402:* 421-425.

[110] Sorra, K.E., & Harris, K.M. (1998). Stability in synapse number and size at 2 hr after long-term potentiation in hippocampal area CA1. *Journal of Neuroscience 18:* 658-671.

[111] Bourgeois, J-P., Goldman-Rakic, P., & Rakic, P. (1999). Formation, elimination and stabilisation of synapses in the primate cerebral cortex. In: M. S. Gazzaniga (Ed.) *Cognitive neuroscience. A handbook for the field,* (2nd edn, pp. 23-32). Cambridge: MIT Press.

[112] Geinisman, Y. (2000). Structural synaptic modifications associated with hippocampal LTP and behavioural learning. *Cerebral Cortex 10:* 952-962.

[113] Fox, C.M., Ramig, L.O., Ciucci, M.R., Sapir, S., McFarland, D. H., Farley, B. G. (2006). The science and practice of LSVT/LOUD: neural plasticity principled approach to treating individuals with Parkinson's disease and other neurological disorders. *Seminars in Speech and Language 27:* 283-299.

[114] Dibble, L.E., Hale, T.F., Marcus, R.L. Gerber, J. P., & LaStayo, P. C. (2009) High intensity eccentric resistance training decreases bradykinesia and improves quality of life in persons with Parkinson's disease: A preliminary study. *Parkinsonism and Related Disorders 15:* 752-757.

[115] Williams, G.P., Morris, M.E. (2009) High-level mobility outcomes following acquired brain injury: A preliminary evaluation. *Brain Injury 23*: 307-312.

INDEX